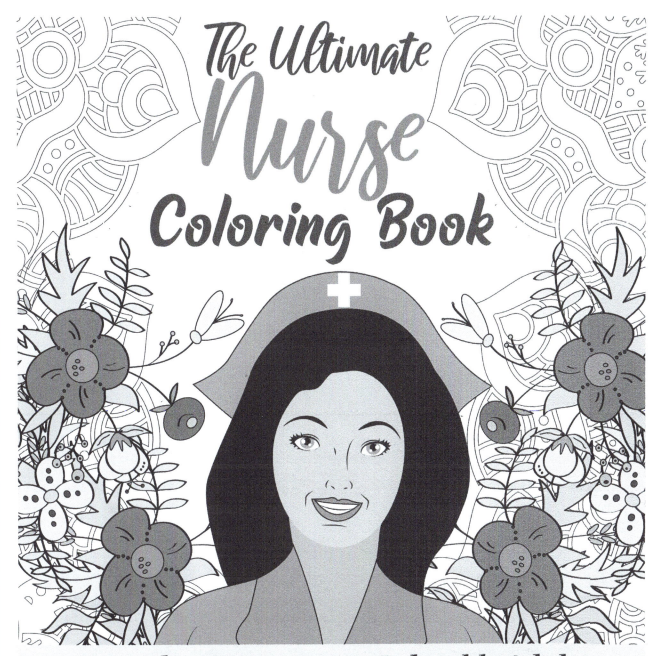

The Ultimate Nurse Coloring Book

A Snarky, Humorous & Relatable Adult Coloring Book for Registered Nurses, Nurse Practitioners and Nursing Students for Stress Relief and Relaxation

Published By Nurse Passion Publishing

This Book Belongs To

_____

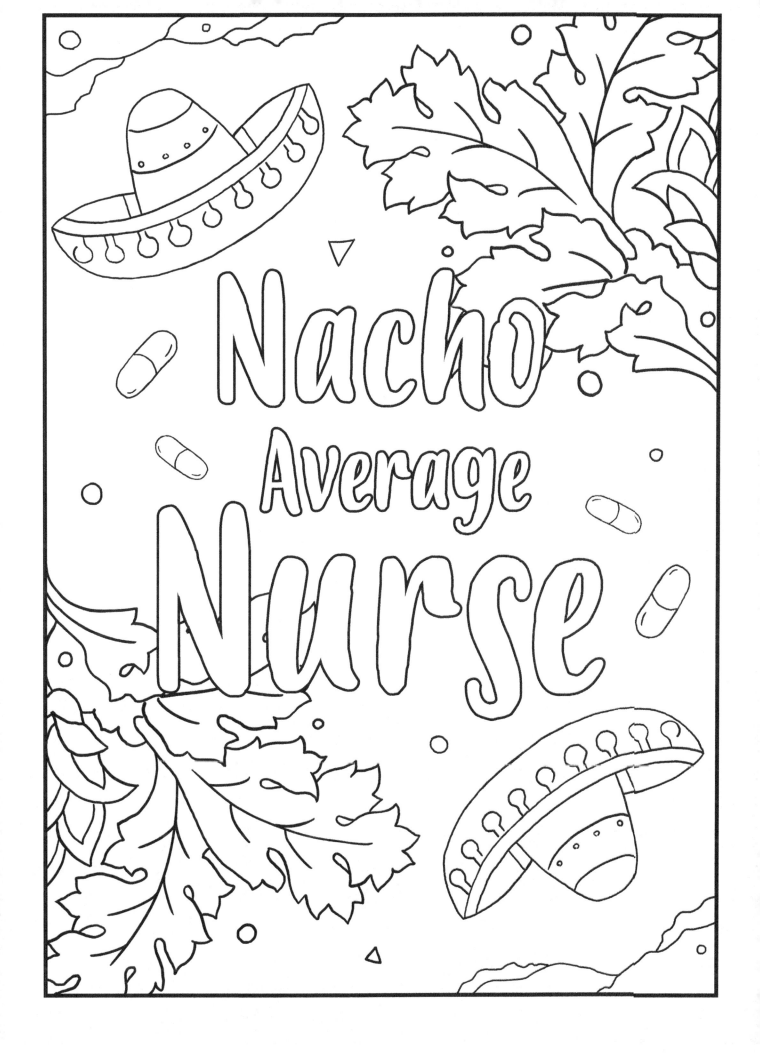

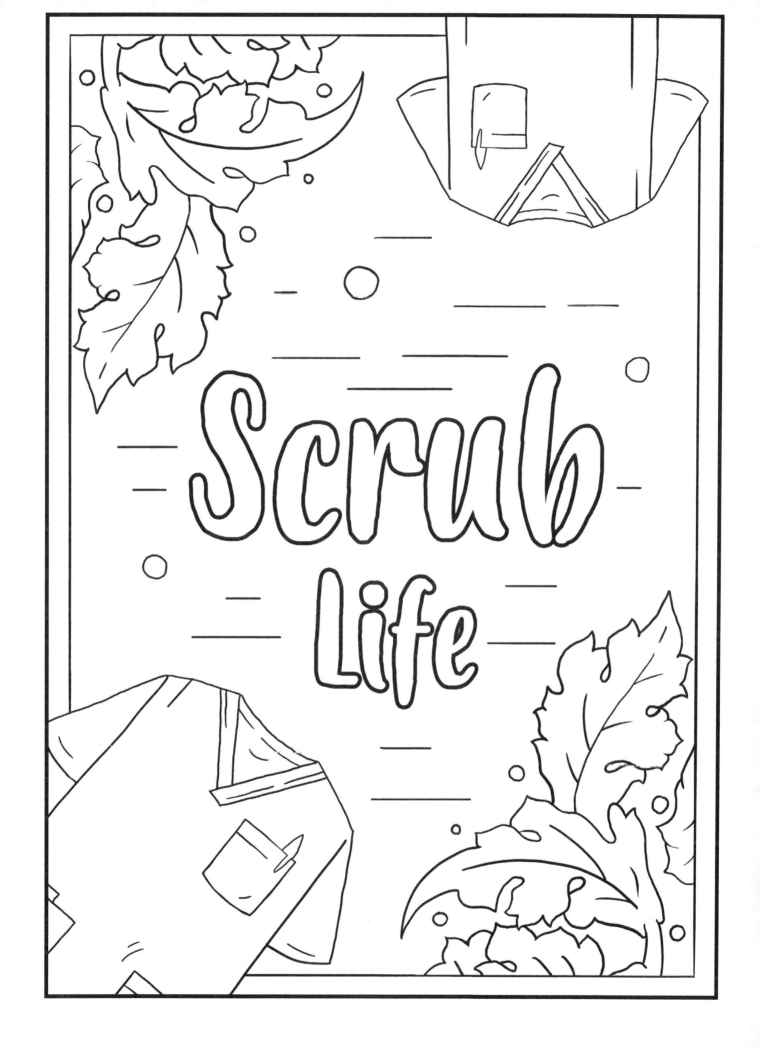

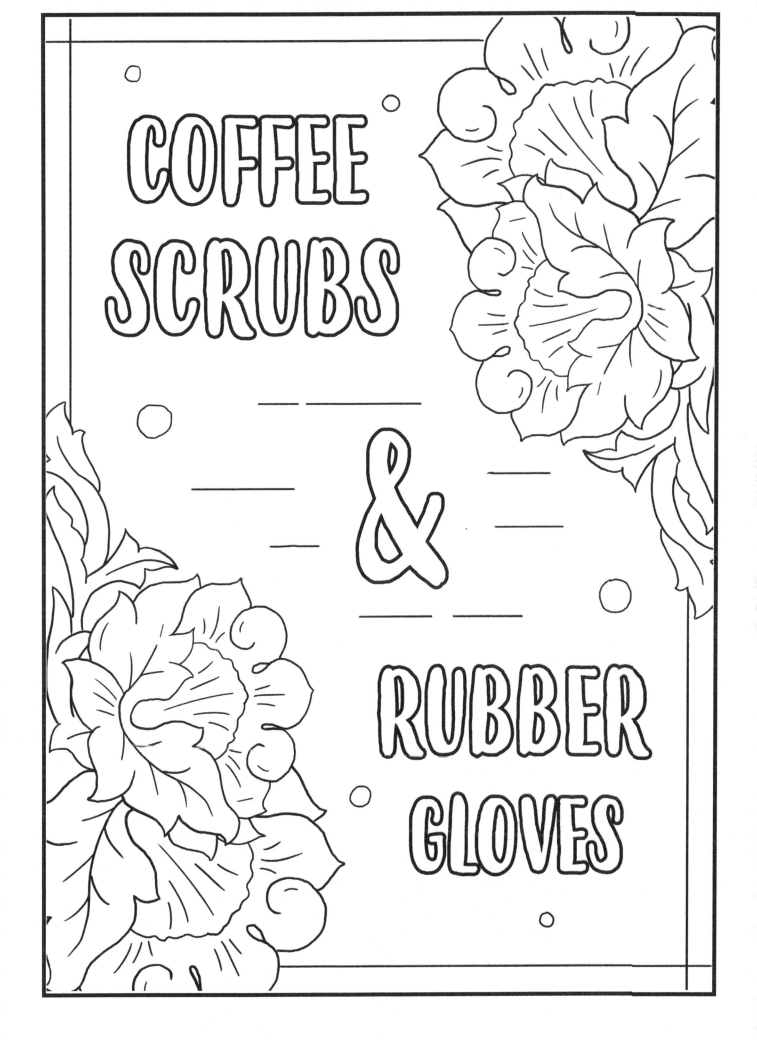

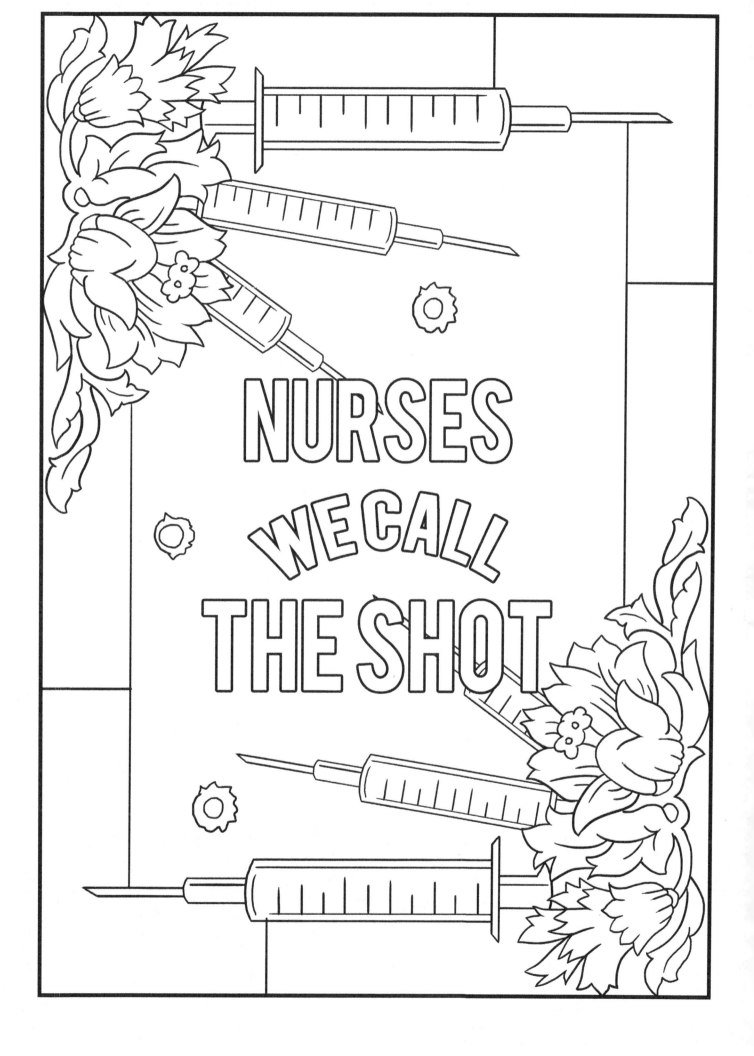

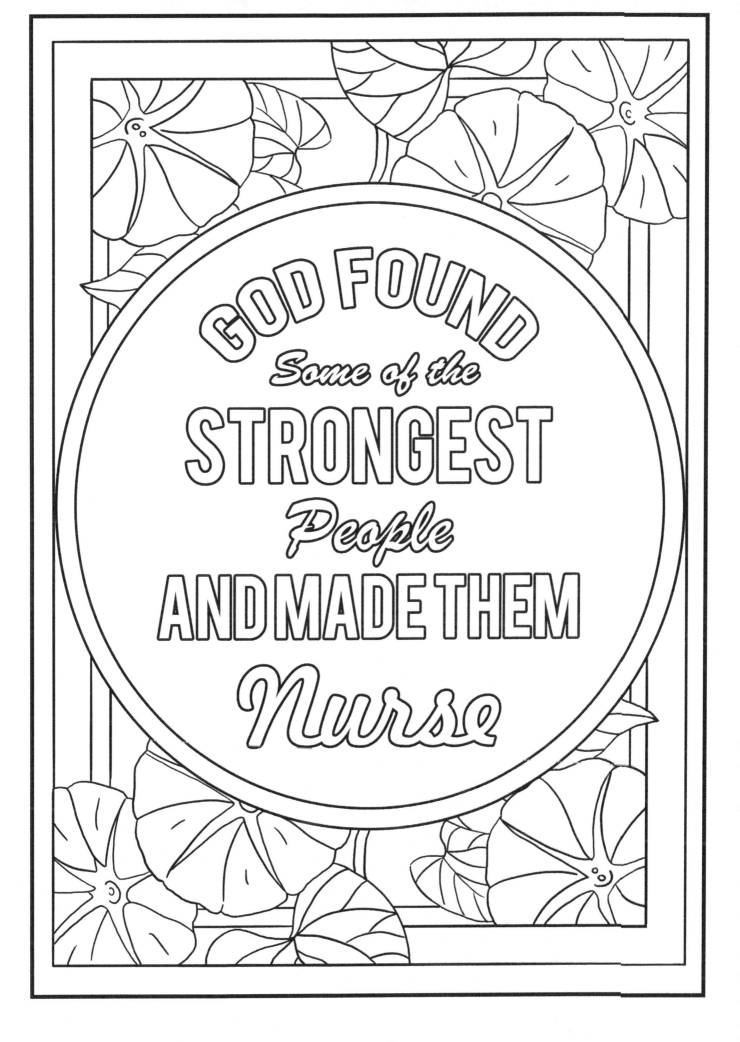

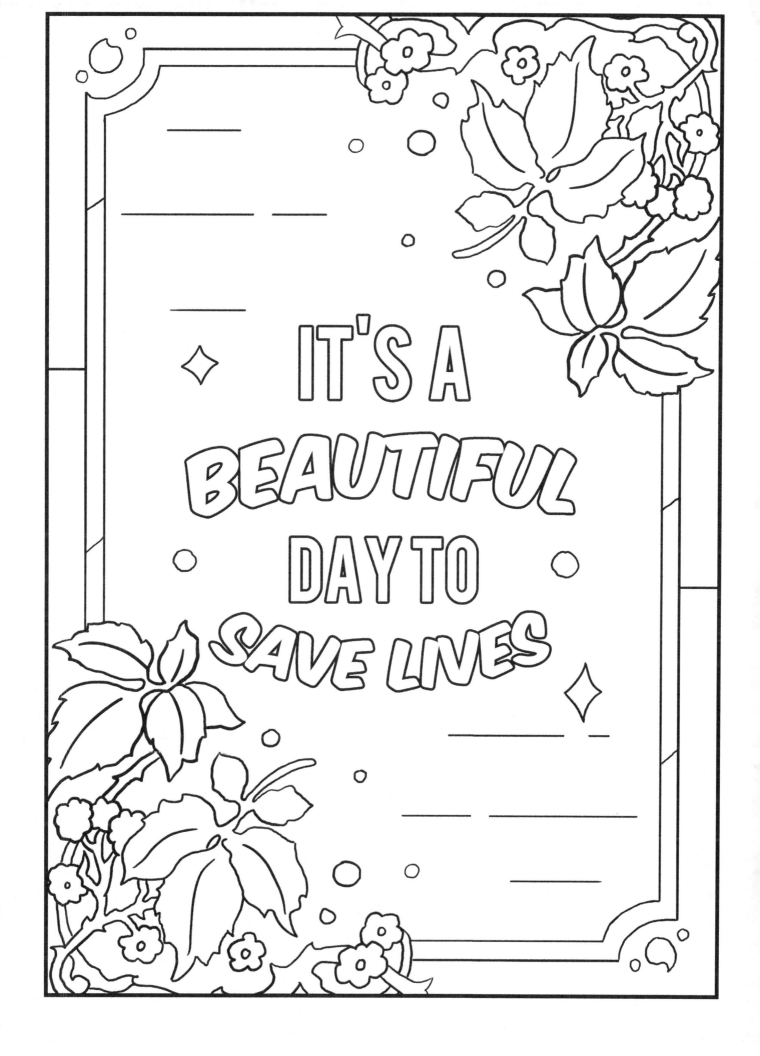

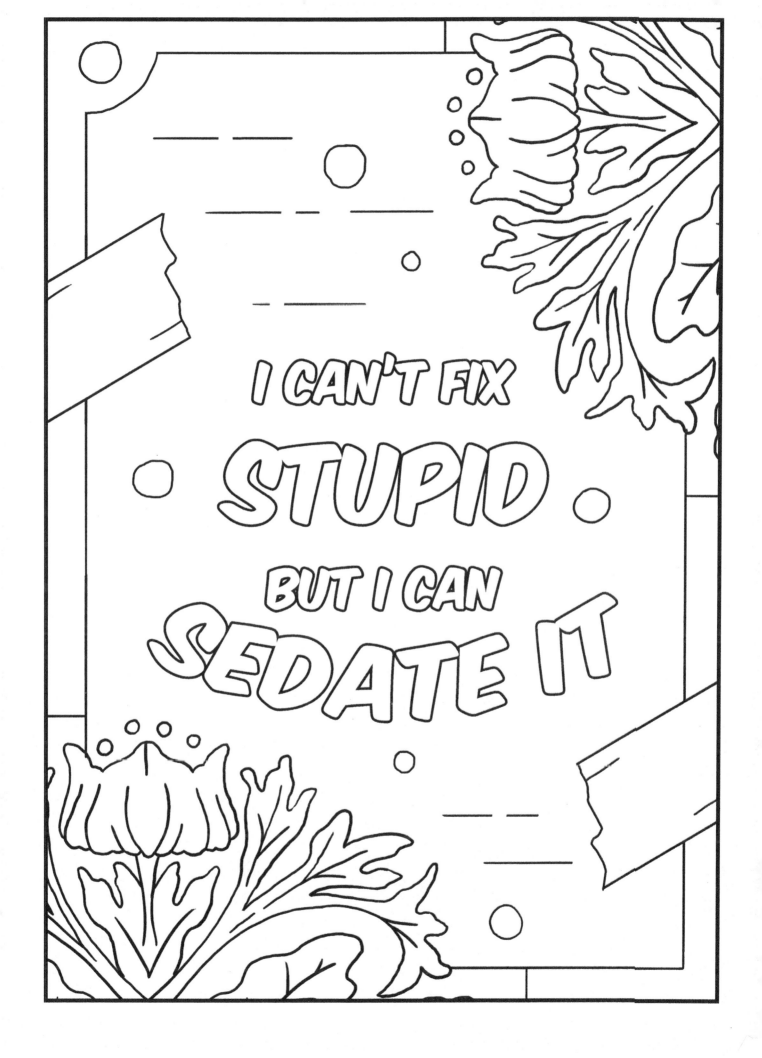

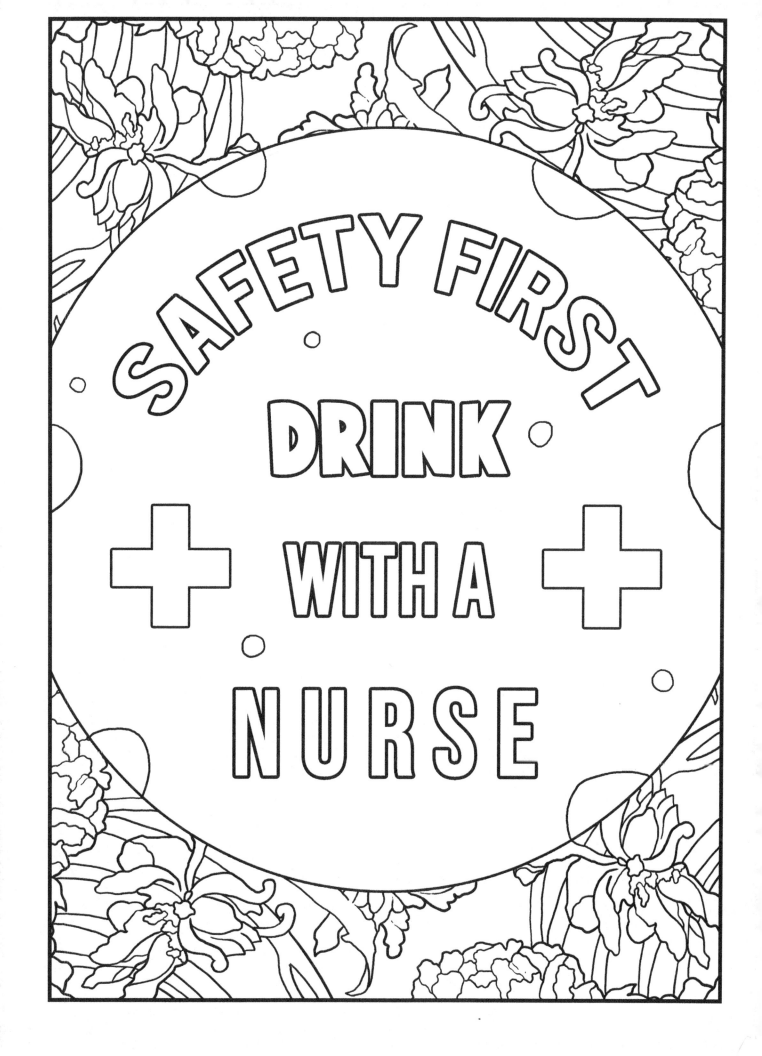

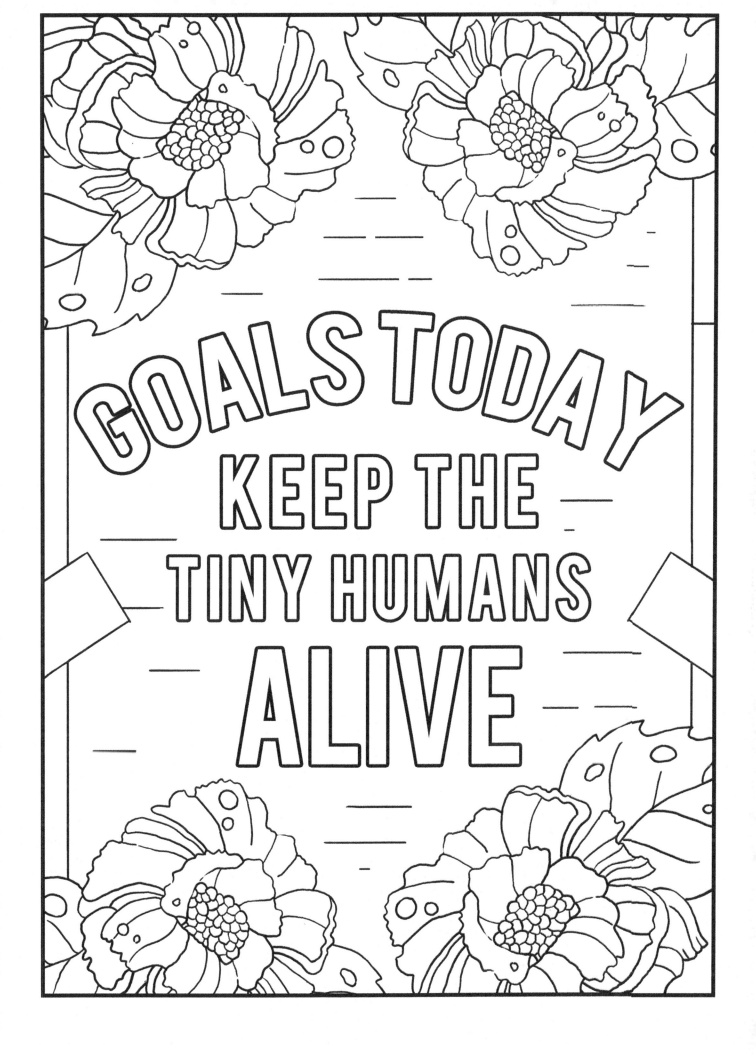

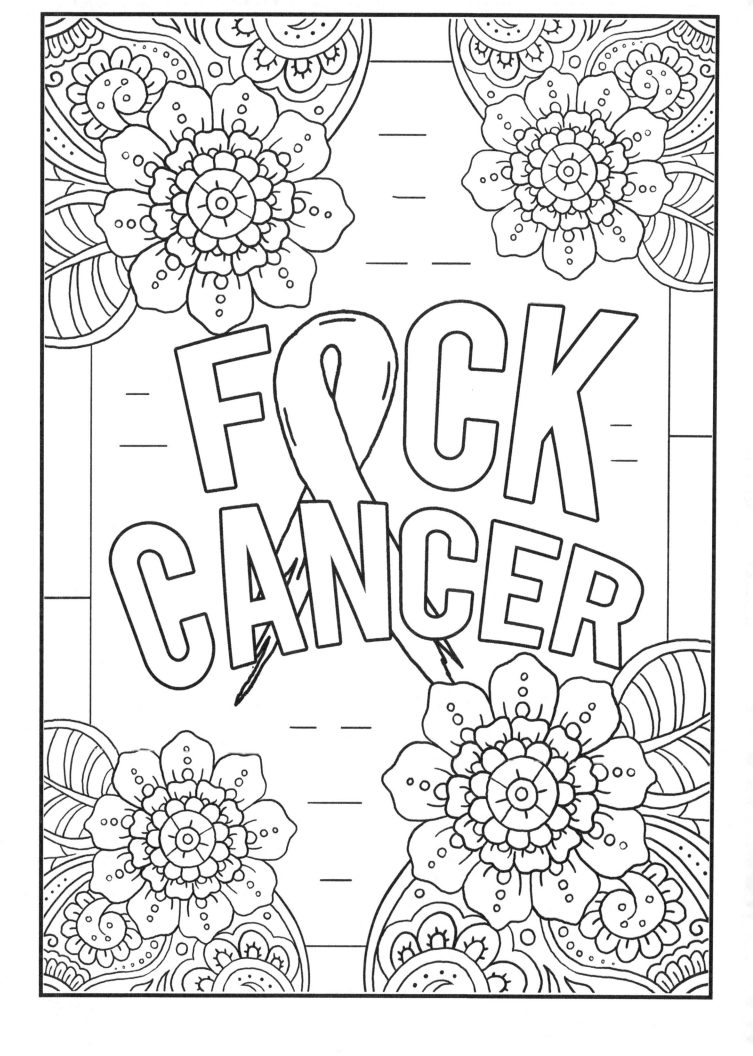

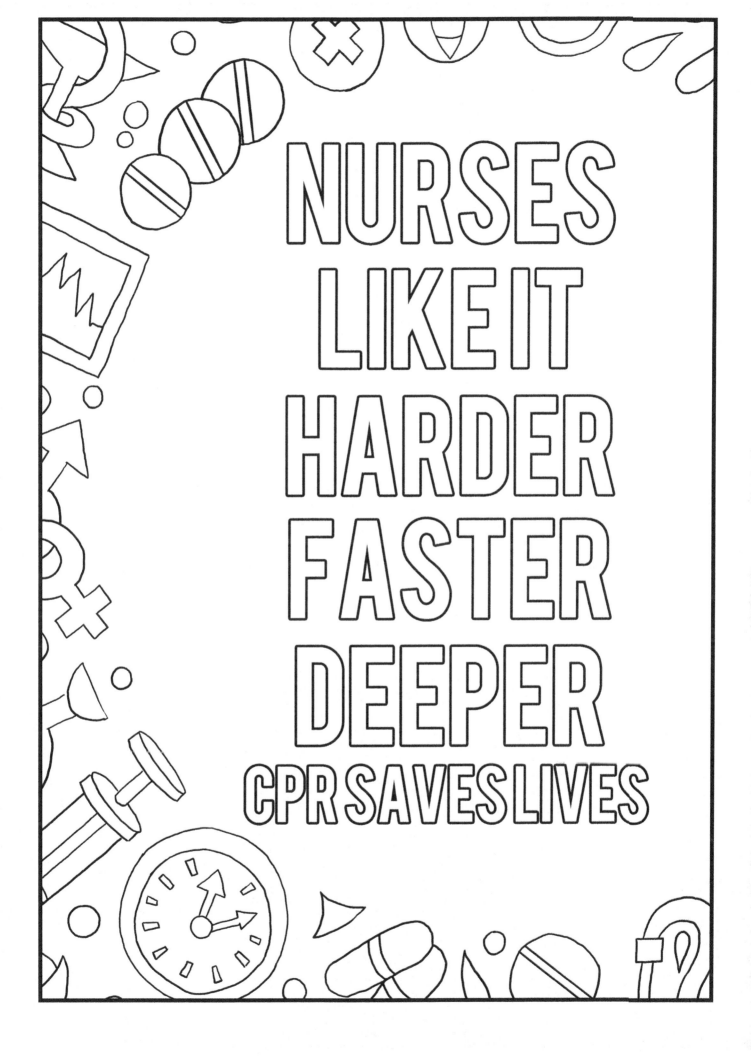

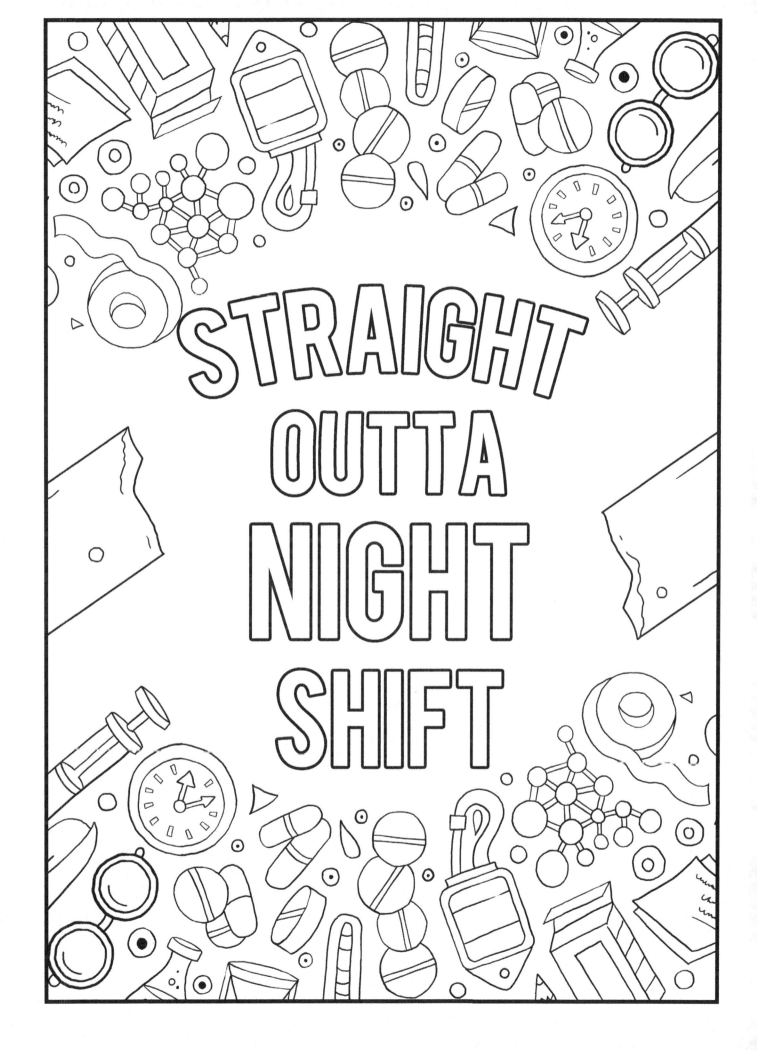

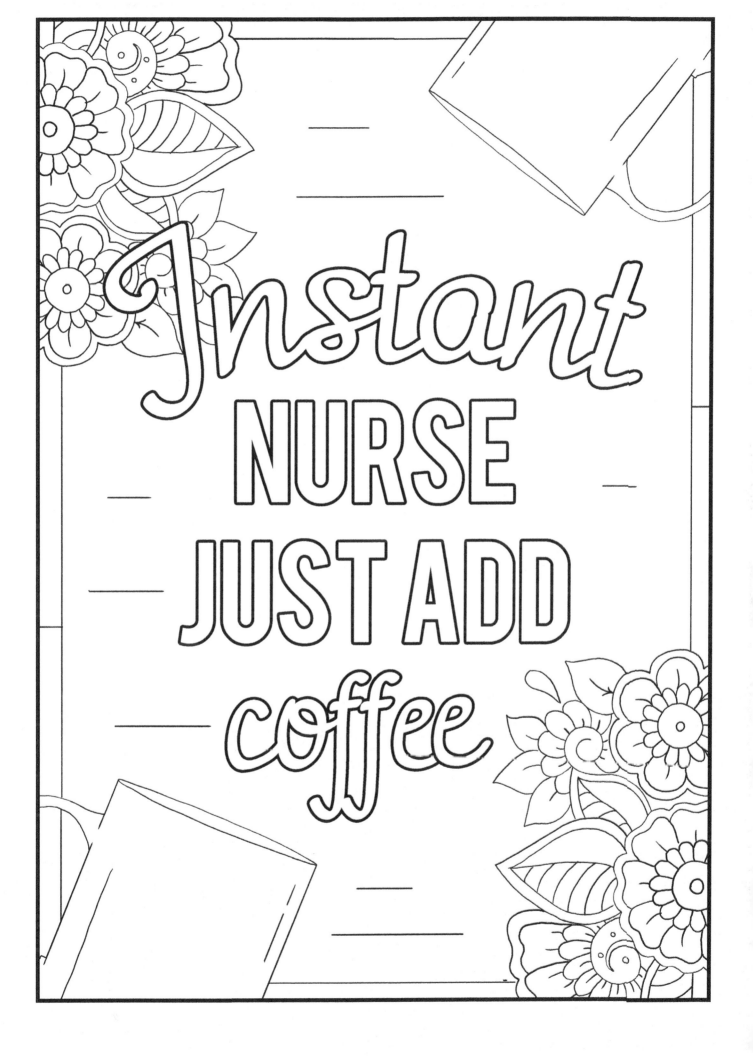

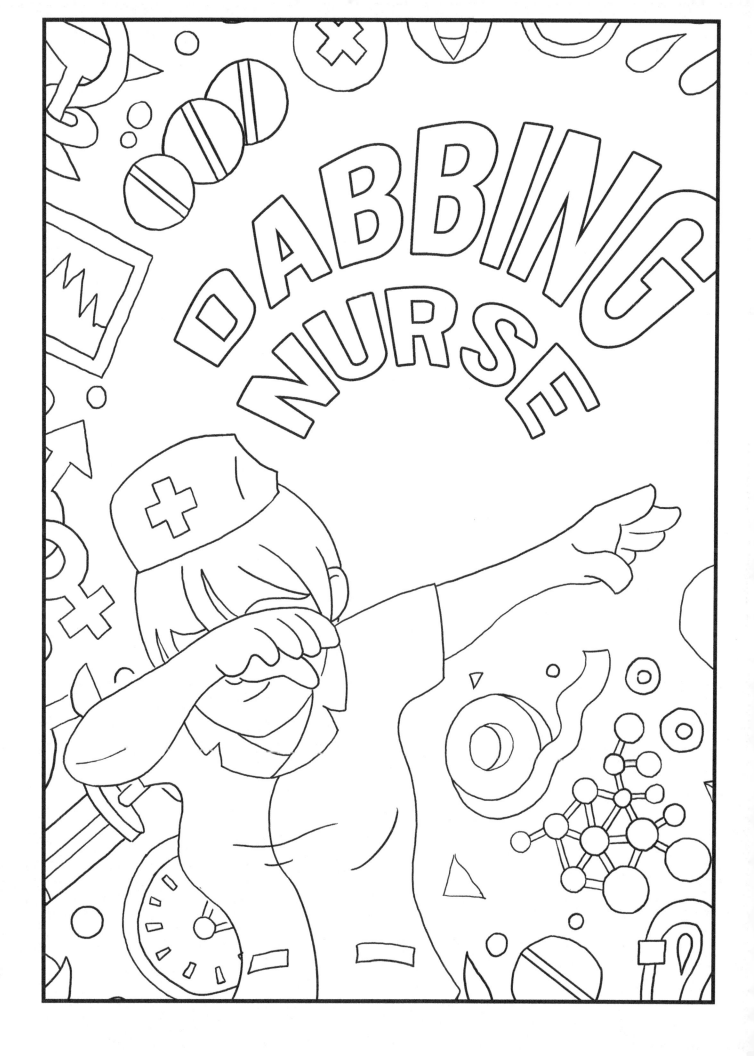

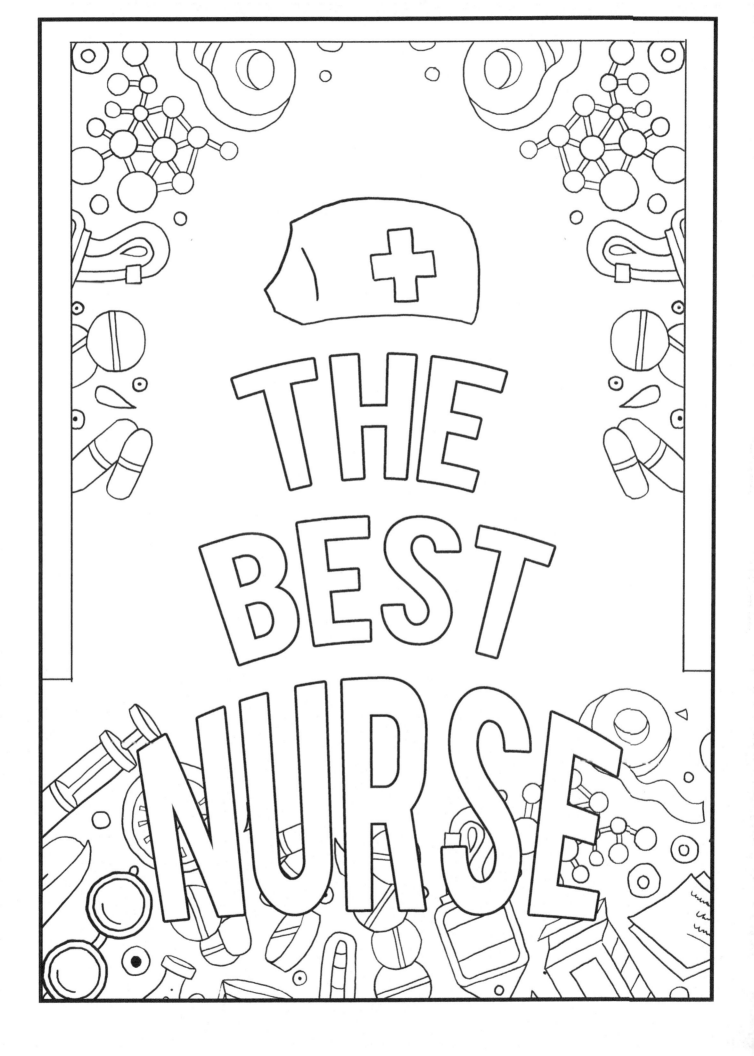

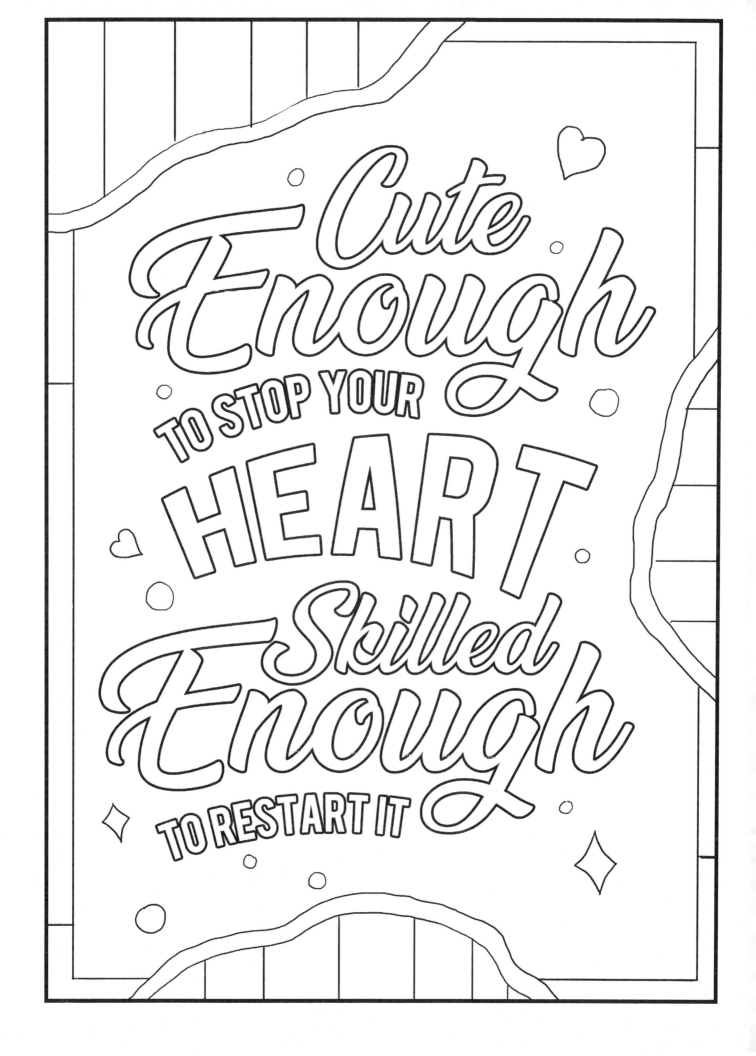

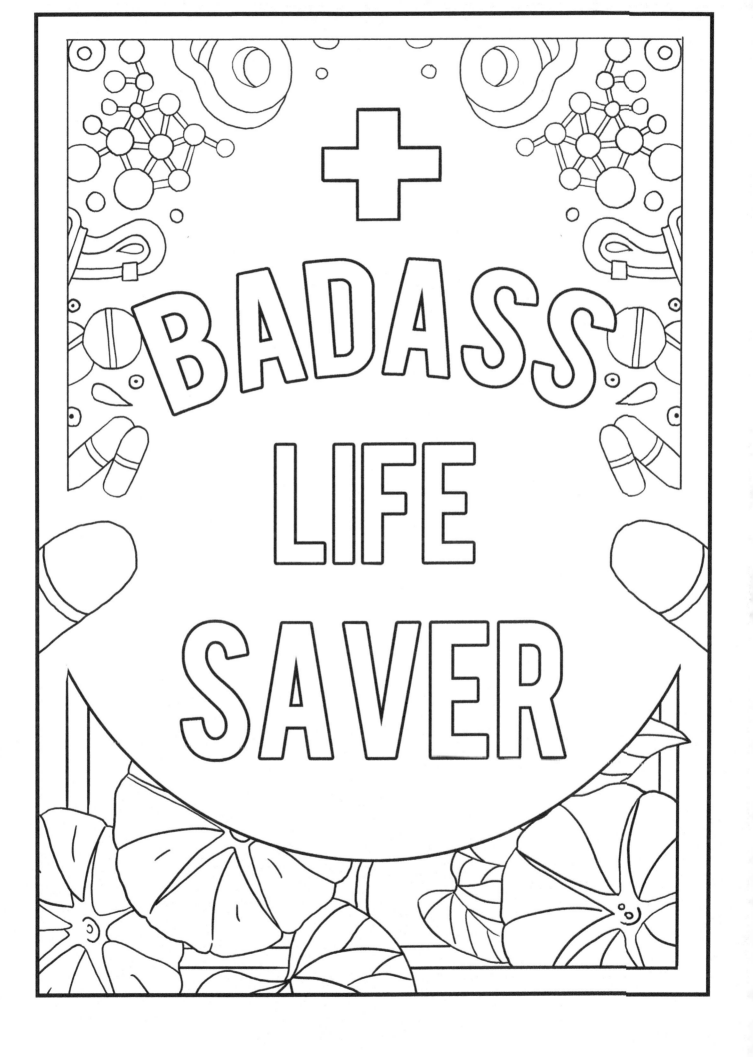

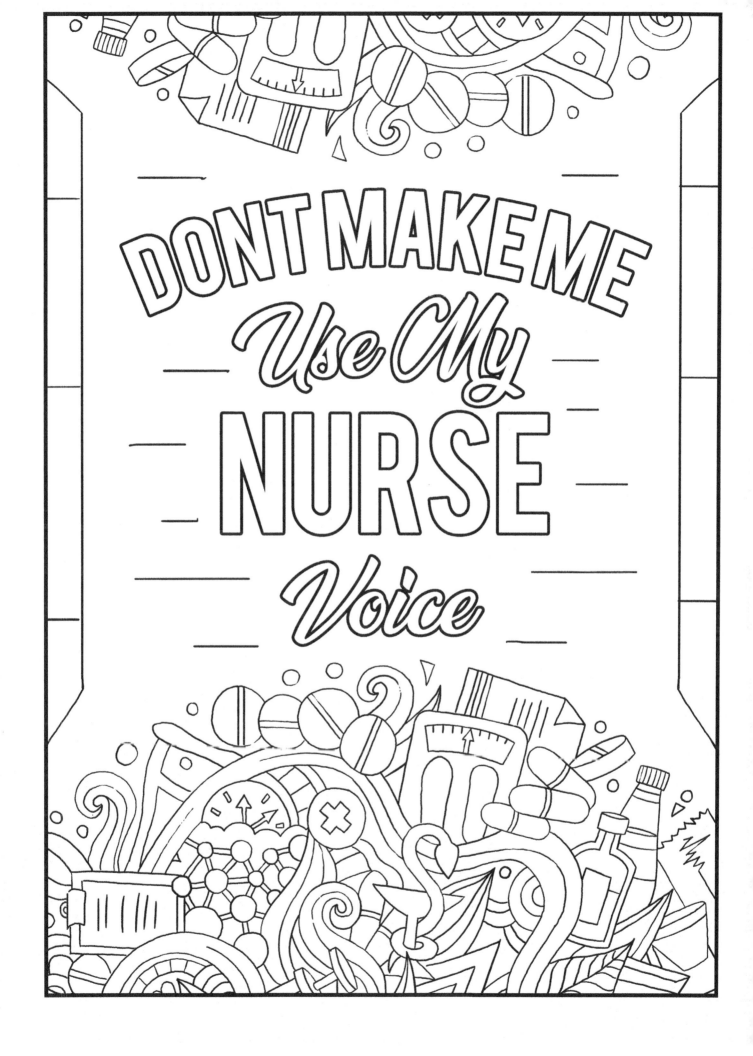

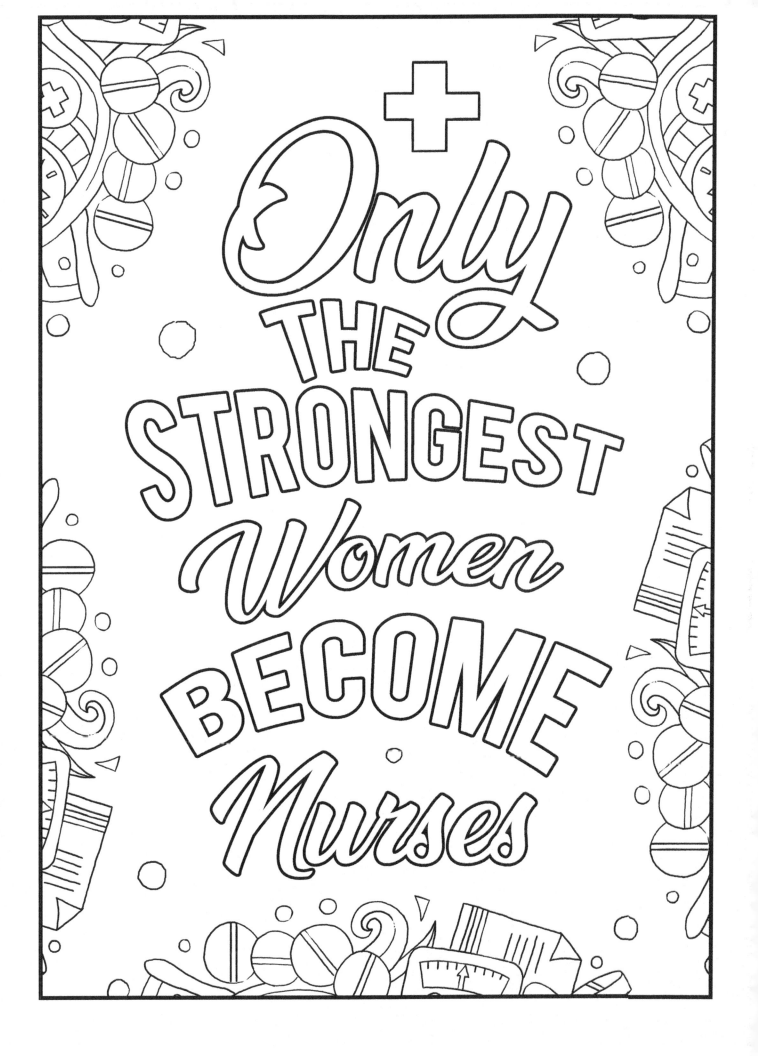

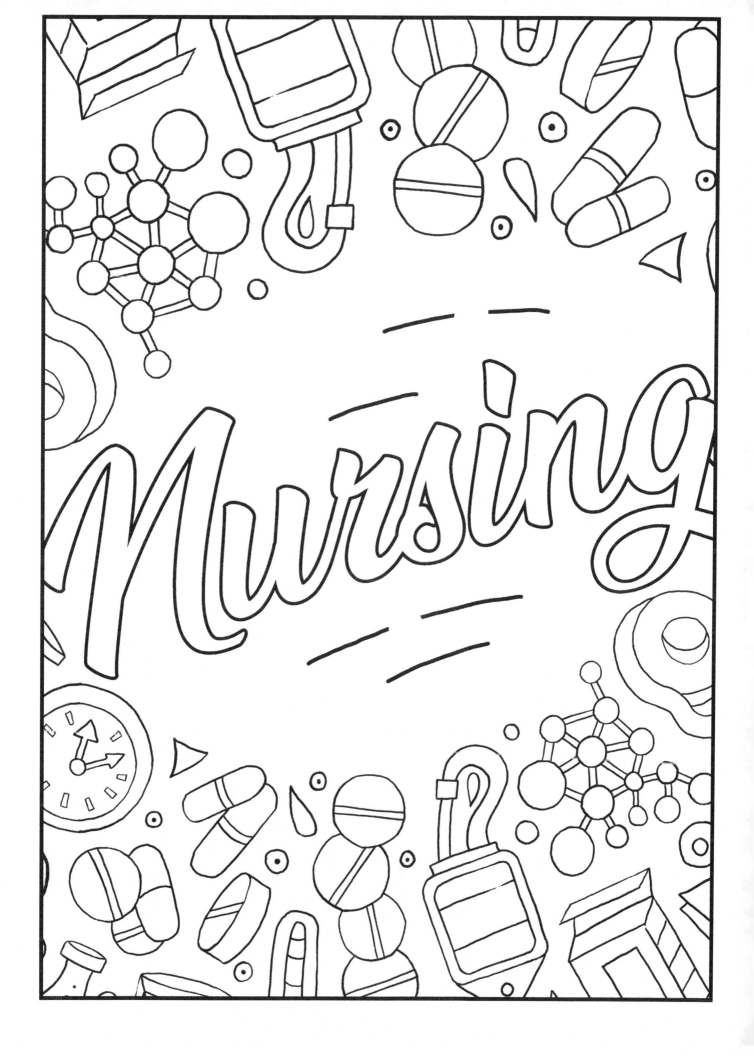

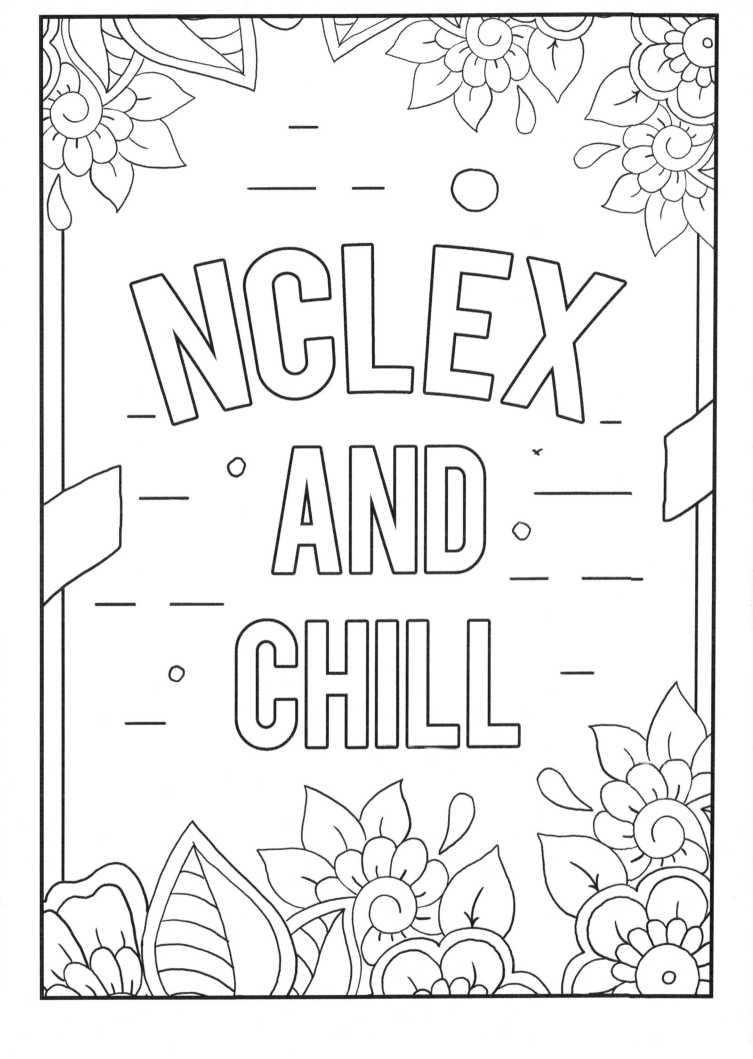

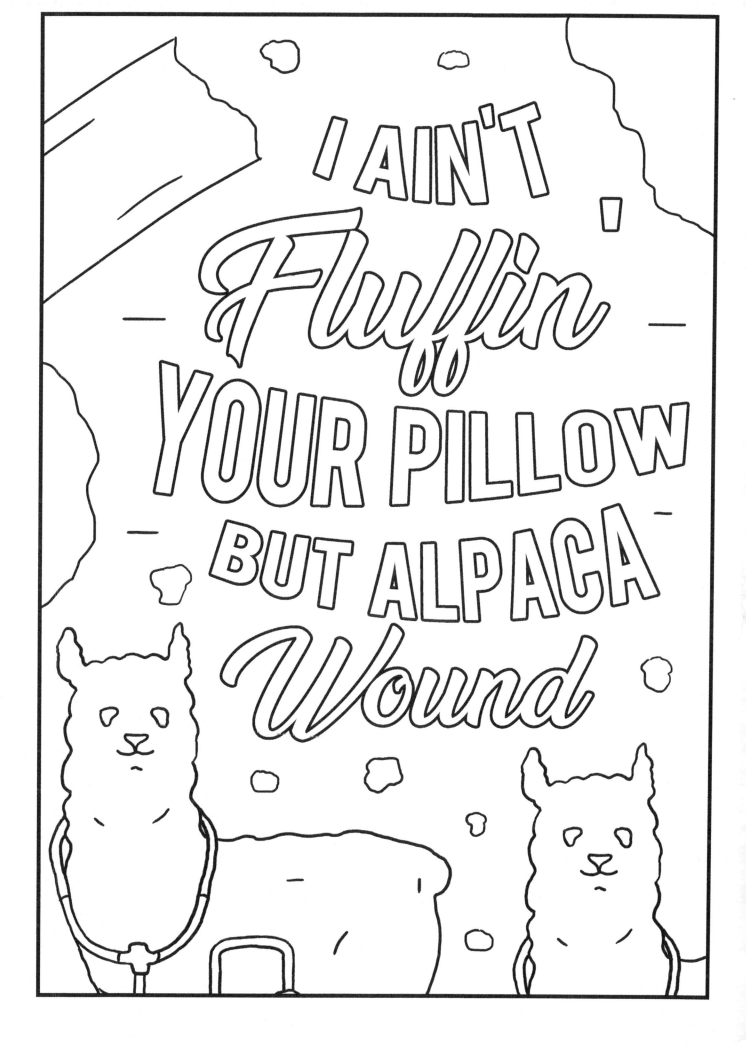

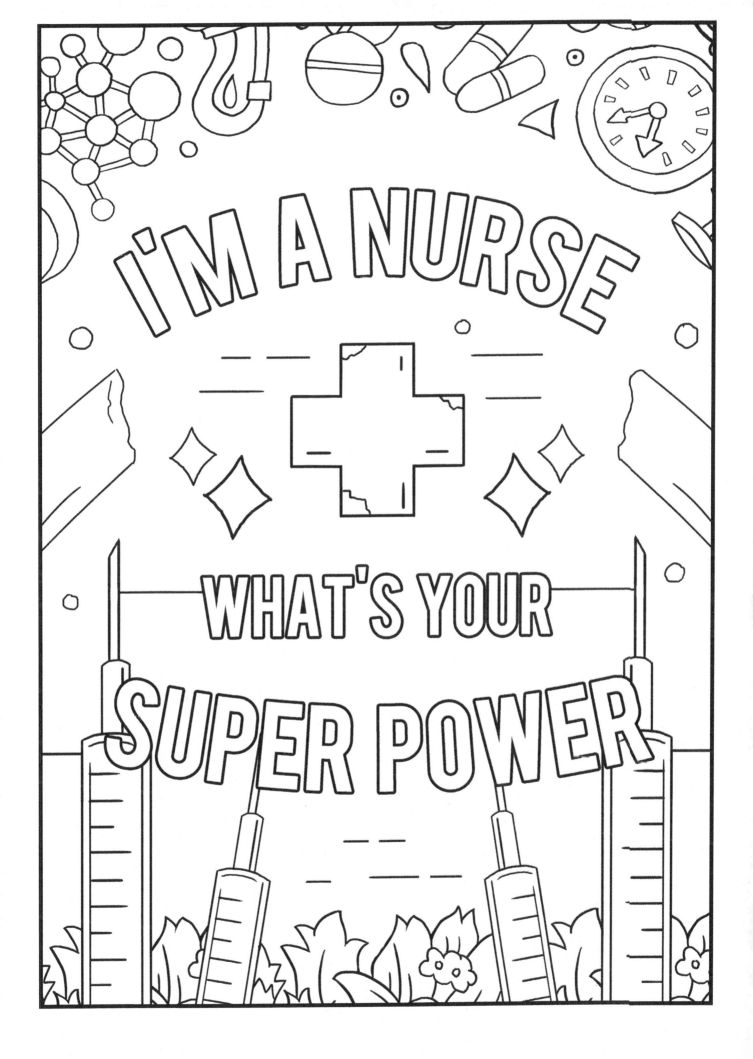

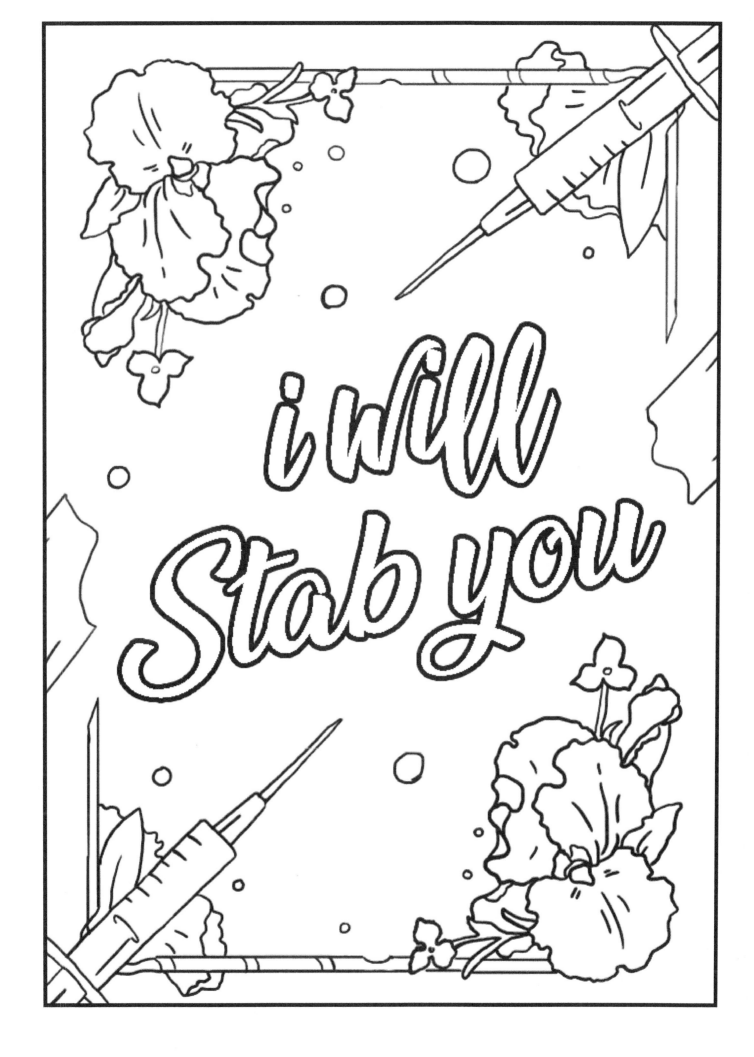

Made in the USA
Coppell, TX
28 February 2020